Essential Air Fryer Recipes

Easy, Delicious and Low Fat Recipes to Master the Full Potential of Your Air Fryer

Dr. Alice Cook

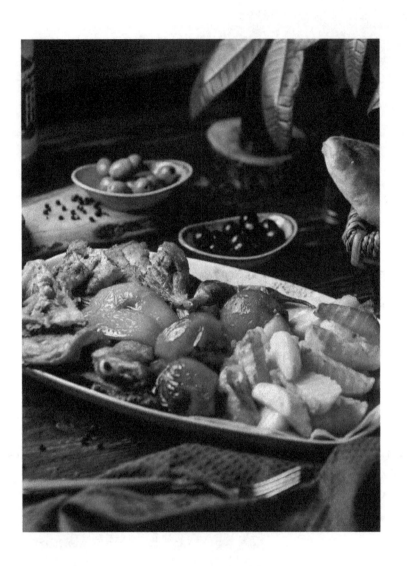

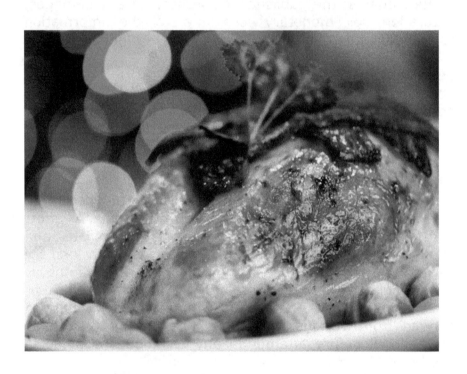

TABLE OF CONTENTS

INTRODUCTION

An Air Fryer is a magic revolutionized kitchen appliance that helps you fry with less or even no oil at all. This kind of product applies Rapid Air technology, which offers a new way on how to fry with less oil. This new invention cooks food through the circulation of superheated air and generates 80% low-fat food. Although the food is fried with less oil, you don't need to worry as the food processed by the Air Fryer still has the same taste as the food that is cooked using the deep-frying method.

This technology uses a superheated element, which radiates heat close to the food and an exhaust fan in its lid to circulate airflow. An Air Fryer ensures that the food processed is cooked completely. The exhaust fan located at the top of the cooking chamber helps the food to get the same heating temperature in every part in short time, resulting to a cooked food of best and healthy quality. Besides, cooking with an Air Fryer is also good for those that are busy and do not have enough time. For example, an Air Fryer only needs half a spoonful of oil and takes 10 minutes to serve a medium bowl of crispy French fries.

In addition to serving healthier food, an Air Fryer also provides some other benefits to you. Since an Air Fryer helps you fry using less oil or without oil at all for some kind of food, it automatically reduces the fat and cholesterol content in food. Surely, no one will refuse to enjoy fried food without worrying about the greasy and fat content. Having fried food with no guilt is really a form of indulging your tongue. Besides having low fat and cholesterol, by consuming oil sparingly, you save some amount of money, which can be used for other needs. An Air Fryer also can reheat your food. Sometimes, when you have fried leftover and you reheat it, it will usually serve reheated greasy food with some addition of unhealthy reuse oil. Surely, the saturated fat in the fried food gets worse because of this process. An Air Fryer helps you reheat your food without being afraid of extra oils that the food may absorb. Fried banana, fish and chips, nuggets, or even fried chicken can be reheated so that they become as warm and crispy as they were before by using an Air Fryer.

Some people may think that spending some amount of

money to buy a fryer is wasteful. I dare to say that they are wrong because actually, an Air Fryer is not only used to fry. It is a sophisticated multi-function appliance since it also helps you to roast chicken, make steak, grill fish, and even bake a cake. With a built-in air filter, an Air Fryer filters the air and saves your kitchen from smoke and grease.

An air Fryer is really a simple innovative method of cooking. Grab it fast and welcome to a clean and healthy kitchen.

Mushrooms and Cheese Spread

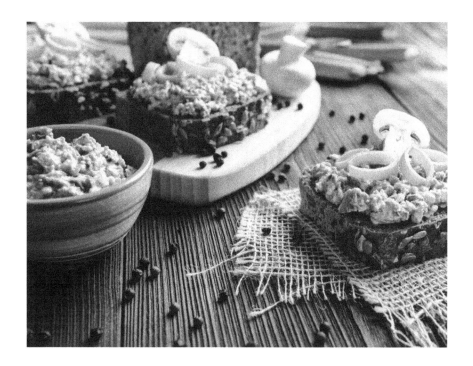

Preparation Time: 25 minutes

Servings: 4

Ingredients:

- ¼ cup mozzarella; shredded
- ½ cup coconut cream
- 1 cup white mushrooms
- A pinch of salt and black pepper

- Cooking spray

Directions:

1. Put the mushrooms in your air fryer's basket, grease with cooking spray and cook at 370°F for 20 minutes.
2. Transfer to a blender, add the remaining ingredients, pulse well, divide into bowls and serve as a spread

Nutrition:

Calories: 202; Fat: 12g; Fiber: 2g; Carbs: 5g; Protein: 7g

Egg, Bacon and Cheese Roll Ups

Preparation Time: 30 minutes

Servings: 4

Ingredients:

- 12 slices sugar-free bacon.
- ½ medium green bell pepper; seeded and chopped
- 6 large eggs.
- ¼ cup chopped onion
- 1 cup shredded sharp Cheddar cheese.
- ½ cup mild salsa, for dipping
- 2 tbsp. unsalted butter.

Directions:

1. In a medium skillet over medium heat, melt butter. Add onion and pepper to the skillet and sauté until fragrant and onions are translucent, about 3 minutes
2. Whisk eggs in a small bowl and pour into skillet. Scramble eggs with onions and peppers until

fluffy and fully cooked, about 5 minutes.
Remove from heat and set aside

3. On work surface, place three slices of bacon side
   by side, overlapping about ¼-inch. Place ¼ cup
   scrambled eggs in a heap on the side closest to
   you and sprinkle ¼ cup cheese on top of the
   eggs.

4. Tightly roll the bacon around the eggs and
   secure the seam with a toothpick if necessary.
   Place each roll into the air fryer basket

5. Adjust the temperature to 350 Degrees F and
   set the timer for 15 minutes. Rotate the rolls
   halfway through the cooking time. Bacon will be
   brown and crispy when completely cooked.
   Serve immediately with salsa for dipping.

Nutrition:

Calories: 460; Protein: 28.2g; Fiber: 0.8g; Fat: 31.7g;
Carbs: 6.1g

Strasbourg Potatoes and Sausages with Curry

Preparation time: 10-20 minutes;

Cooking time: 15-30 minutes;

Serve: 6

Ingredients:

- 750 g of fresh potatoes
- 3 Strasbourg sausages
- 2 small spoons of curry
- Salt to taste

Direction:

1. Peel the potatoes and cut them into cubes of approximately 1 cm per side. Put the Perl apples to soak in water, drain them and dry them well with a paper towel.
2. After spraying the air fryer with cooking spray, pour potatoes, salt.
3. Set the temperature to 150°C and simmer the potatoes for 20 minutes.

4. Add the Strasbourg sausages cut into small pieces, curry, and cook for another 10 minutes.

Nutrition:

Calories 418.5, Fat 17.6 g, Carbohydrate 42.1 g, Sugars 2.1 g, Protein 18.0 g, Cholesterol44.5 mg

Air Fryer Breakfast Casserole

Preparation Time: 10 minutes

Cooking Time: 25 minutes

Servings: 2

Ingredients:

- 3 red potatoes
- 3 eggs
- 2 turkey sausage patties
- ¼ cup cheddar cheese
- 1 tablespoon milk
- Olive oil cooking spray

Directions:

1. Preheat the Air fryer to 400 ° F and grease a baking dish with cooking spray.
2. Place the potatoes in the Air fryer basket and cook for about 10 minutes.
3. Whisk eggs with milk in a bowl.
4. Put the potatoes and sausage in the baking dish and pour egg mixture on top.

5. Sprinkle with cheddar cheese and arrange in the Air fryer.

6. Cook for about 15 minutes at 350 ° F and dish out to serve warm.

Nutrition:

Calories: 469, Fat: 16.3g, Carbohydrates: 51.9g, Sugar: 4.1g, Protein: 29.1g, Sodium: 623mg

Cod Tortilla

Preparation Time: 27 minutes

Servings: 4

Ingredients:

- 4 cod fillets; skinless and boneless
- 4 tortillas
- 1 green bell pepper; chopped.
- 1 red onion; chopped.
- A drizzle of olive oil
- 1 cup corn
- 1/2 cup salsa
- 4 tbsp. parmesan cheese; grated
- A handful of baby spinach

Directions:

1. Put the fish fillets in your air fryer's basket, cook at 350°F for 6 minutes and transfer to a plate.
2. Heat up a pan with the oil over medium heat, add the bell peppers, onions and corn and stir
3. Sauté for 5 minutes and take off the heat.

Arrange all the tortillas on a working surface and divide the cod, salsa, sautéed veggies, spinach and parmesan evenly between the 4 tortillas; then wrap / roll them

4. Place the tortillas in your air fryer's basket and cook at 350°F for 6 minutes. Divide between plates, serve.

Carrot Oatmeal

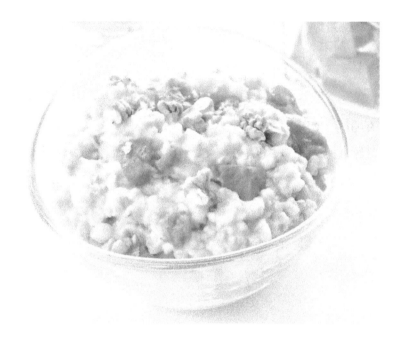

Preparation Time: 20 minutes

Servings: 4

Ingredients:

- 1/2 cup steel cut oats
- 2 cups almond milk
- 1 cup carrots; shredded
- 2 tsp. sugar

- 1 tsp. cardamom; ground
- Cooking spray

Directions:

1. Spray your air fryer with cooking spray, add all ingredients, toss and cover. Cook at 365°F for 15 minutes. Divide into bowls and serve

Green Beans

Preparation Time: 25 minutes

Servings: 4

Ingredients:

- 6 cups green beans; trimmed
- 1 tbsp. hot paprika
- 2 tbsp. olive oil
- A pinch of salt and black pepper

Directions:

1. Take a bowl and mix the green beans with the other ingredients, toss, put them in the air fryer's basket and cook at 370°F for 20 minutes
2. Divide between plates and serve as a side dish.

Nutrition:

Calories: 120; Fat: 5g; Fiber: 1g; Carbs: 4g; Protein: 2g

Bok Choy and Butter Sauce

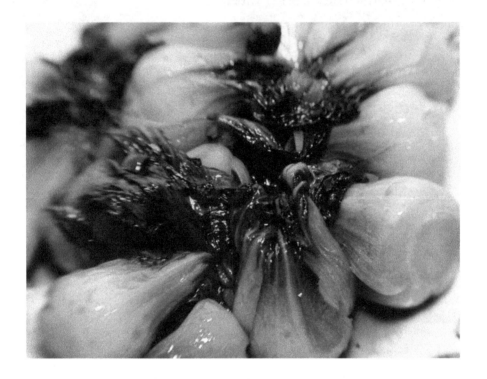

Preparation Time: 20 minutes

Servings: 4

Ingredients:

- 2 bok choy heads; trimmed and cut into strips
- 1 tbsp. butter; melted
- 2 tbsp. chicken stock

- 1 tsp. lemon juice

- 1 tbsp. olive oil

- A pinch of salt and black pepper

Directions:

1. In a pan that fits your air fryer, mix all the ingredients, toss, introduce the pan in the air fryer and cook at 380°F for 15 minutes.

2. Divide between plates and serve as a side dish

Nutrition:

Calories: 141; Fat: 3g; Fiber: 2g; Carbs: 4g; Protein: 3g

Creamy Fennel

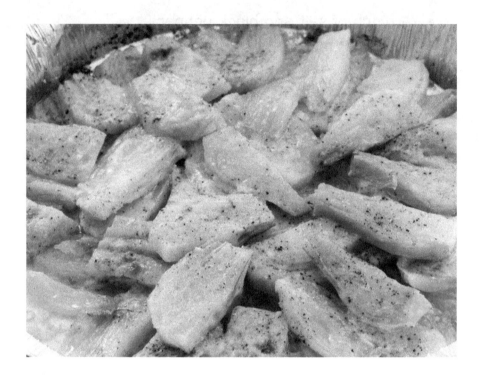

Preparation Time: 17 minutes

Servings: 4

Ingredients:

- 2 big fennel bulbs; sliced
- ½ cup coconut cream
- 2 tbsp. butter; melted

- Salt and black pepper to taste.

Directions:

1. In a pan that fits the air fryer, combine all the ingredients, toss, introduce in the machine and cook at 370°F for 12 minutes

2. Divide between plates and serve as a side dish.

Nutrition:

Calories: 151; Fat: 3g; Fiber: 2g; Carbs: 4g; Protein: 6g

Yummy Potatoes Gratin

Preparation Time: 55 minutes

Servings: 3

Ingredients:

- 7 medium russet potatoes; peeled
- 1/2 cup milk
- 1/2 cup cream
- 1 teaspoon black pepper
- 1/2 teaspoon nutmeg
- 1/2 cup Gruyère or semi-mature cheese; grated

Directions:

1. Preheat the Air Fryer to 390 - degrees Fahrenheit.
2. Slice the potatoes wafer-thin. In a bowl; mix the milk and cream and season to taste with salt, pepper and nutmeg.
3. Coat the potato slices with the milk mixture.
4. Transfer the potato slices to 8-inch heat resistant baking dish and pour the rest of the

cream mixture from the bowl on top of the potatoes.

5. Place the baking dish in the cooking basket into the Air Fryer.

6. Set the timer and cook for 25 minutes. Remove cooking basket and distribute the cheese evenly over the potatoes.

7. Set the timer for 10 minutes and bake the gratin until it is nicely browned.

8. Tips: Instead of milk you can substitute two eggs

Rosemary Potato Chips

Preparation Time: 1 hour 15 minutes

Servings: 2

Ingredients:

- 4 medium russet potatoes
- 1 tablespoon olive oil
- 2 teaspoon rosemary; chopped
- 2 pinches salt

Directions:

1. Scrub the potatoes under running water to clean.
2. Cut the potatoes lengthwise and peel them into thin chips directly into a mixing bowl full of water.
3. Soak the potatoes for 30 minutes; changing the water several times. Drain thoroughly and pat completely dry with a paper towel.
4. Preheat the Air Fryer to 330 - degrees Fahrenheit. In a mixing bowl; toss the potatoes

with olive oil. Place them into the cooking basket and cook for 30 minutes or until golden brown, shaking frequently to ensure the chips are cooked evenly.

5. When finished and still warm, toss in a large bowl with rosemary and salt.

Roasted Brussels Sprouts

Preparation Time: 30 minutes

Servings: 3

Ingredients:

- 2 cups Brussels sprouts
- 1/4 cup pine nuts [toasted]
- 1 orange [juice and zest]
- 1/4 raisins [drained]
- 1 tablespoon oil [olive]

Directions:

1. Preheat Air Fryer to 390 – degrees Fahrenheit.
2. Boil sprouts for about 4 minutes and then put them in cold water and drain the sprouts properly.
3. Meanwhile; soak raisins in orange juice for 15 minutes. Now roast the cooled sprouts with oil for 15 minutes. Serve with nuts, raisins and zest.

Air-Fried Crab Sticks

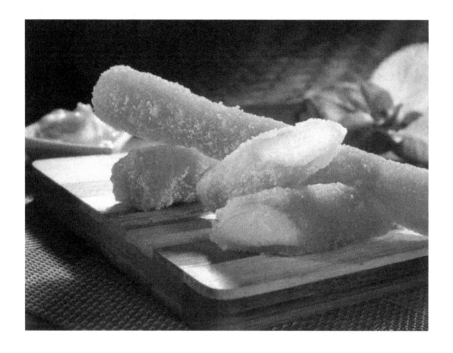

Preparation time: 10 minutes

Servings: 2-3

Ingredients:

- Crab sticks: 1 package
- Cooking oil spray: as needed

Directions:

1. Take each of the sticks out of the package and unroll until flat. Tear the sheets into thirds.

2. Arrange them on a plate and lightly spritz using cooking spray. Set the timer for 10 minutes.

3. Note: If you shred the crab meat; you can cut the time in half, but they will also easily fall through the holes in the basket.

Breaded Cod Sticks

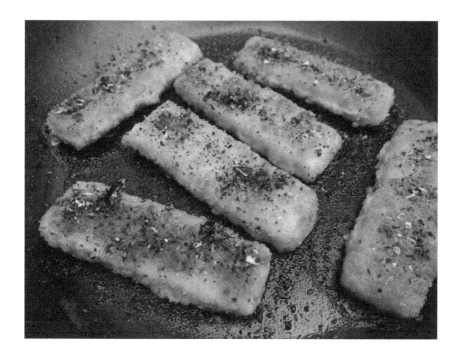

Preparation time: 15 minutes

Servings: 5

Ingredients:

- Milk: 3 tbsp.
- Large eggs: 2
- Breadcrumbs: 2 cups
- Salt: .25 tsp.

- Black pepper: .5 tsp.
- Almond flour: 1 cup
- Cod: 1 lb.

Directions:

1. Set the Air Fryer at 350º Fahrenheit.
2. Prepare three bowls; 1 with the milk and eggs; 1 with the pepper, salt, and breadcrumbs; and another with almond flour.
3. Dip the sticks in the flour, egg mixture, and lastly - the breadcrumbs.
4. Arrange in the basket and set the timer for 12 minutes – shaking halfway through the cooking process.
5. Serve with your favorite sauce.

Fish & Chips

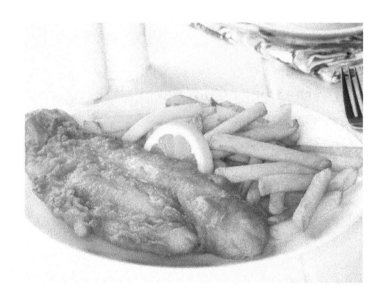

Preparation time: 10 minutes

Servings: 4

Ingredients:

- Catfish fillets or similar fish: 2
- Wholemeal bread for breadcrumbs: 3 slices
- Medium beaten egg: 1
- Bag tortilla chips: 0.88 oz. or approximately/25g
- Juice and rind of 1 lemon

- Pepper and salt
- Parsley: 1 tbsp.

Directions:

1. Warm the fryer before baking time to reach 356° Fahrenheit.
2. Zest and juice the lemon.
3. Slice the fillets into four pieces ready for cooking. Season each one with the lemon juice and set aside for a few minutes.
4. Use a food processor to mix the tortillas, parsley, pepper, breadcrumbs, and lemon zest.
5. Whisk the egg and egg wash the fish. Run it through the crumb mixture. Place them onto the baking tray and cook until crispy.
6. Preparation time is ten minutes with a total cooking time of fifteen minutes; so, wait patiently to enjoy.

Shrimp and Spaghetti

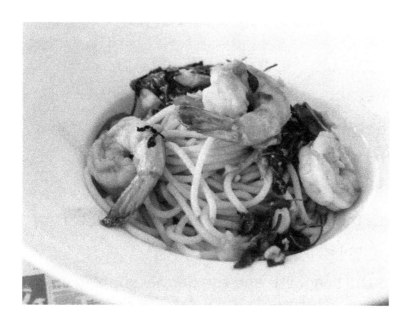

Preparation Time: 20 minutes

Servings: 4

Ingredients:

- 1 lb. shrimp; cooked, peeled and deveined
- 10 oz. canned tomatoes; chopped.
- 1 cup parmesan cheese; grated
- 2 tbsp. olive oil
- 1/4 tsp. oregano; dried

- 12 oz. spaghetti; cooked
- 1 garlic clove; minced
- 1 tbsp. parsley; finely chopped.

Directions:

1. In a pan that fits your air fryer, add the shrimp with the oil, garlic, tomatoes, oregano and parsley; toss well.
2. Place the pan in the fryer and cook at 380°F for 10 minutes
3. Add the spaghetti and the parmesan; toss well. Divide between plates, serve and enjoy!

Chicken with Carrots

Preparation Time: 15 minutes

Cooking Time: 25 minutes

Servings: 2

- **Ingredients:**
- 1 carrot, peeled and thinly sliced
- 2 tablespoons butter
- 2: 4-ounceschicken breast halves
- 1 tablespoon fresh rosemary, chopped
- Salt and black pepper, as required
- 2 tablespoons fresh lemon juice

Directions:

1. Preheat the Air fryer to 375 degree F and grease an Air fryer basket.
2. Place 2 square-shaped parchment papers onto a smooth surface and arrange carrot slices evenly in the center of each parchment paper.
3. Drizzle ½ tablespoon of butter over carrot slices and season with salt and black pepper.

4. Layer with chicken breasts and top with rosemary, lemon juice and remaining butter.

5. Fold the parchment paper on all sides and transfer into the Air fryer.

6. Cook for about 25 minutes and dish out in a serving platter to serve.

Nutrition:

Calories: 339, Fats: 20.3g, Carbohydrates: 4.4g, Sugar: 1.8g, Proteins: 33.4g, Sodium: 2822mg

Rosemary Chicken Breasts

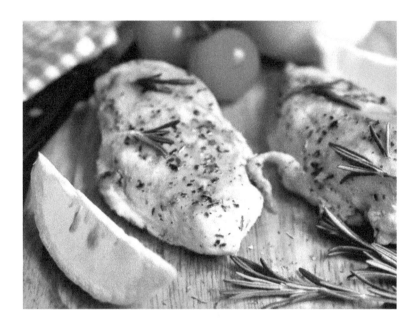

Preparation Time: 35 minutes

Servings: 4

Ingredients:

- 2 chicken breasts; skinless, boneless and halved
- 1 yellow onion; sliced
- 1 cup chicken stock
- 4 garlic cloves; chopped.
- 2 tbsp. cornstarch mixed with 2½ tbsp. water

- 2 tbsp. butter; melted
- 1 tbsp. soy sauce
- 1 tsp. rosemary; dried
- 1 tbsp. fresh rosemary; chopped.
- Salt and black pepper to taste

Directions:

1. Heat up the butter in a pan that fits your air fryer over medium heat.
2. Add the onions, garlic, dried and fresh rosemary, stock, soy sauce, salt and pepper; stir and simmer for 2-3 minutes
3. Add the cornstarch mixture, whisk, cook for 2 minutes more and take off the heat
4. Add the chicken, toss gently and place the pan in the fryer; cook at 370°F for 20 minutes. Divide between plates and serve hot.

Duck Breast and Potatoes

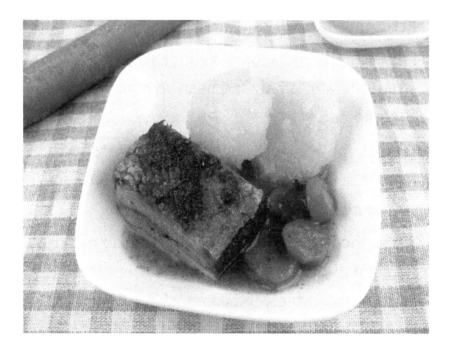

Preparation Time: 40 minutes

Servings: 2

Ingredients:

- 1 duck breast; halved and scored
- 1 oz. red wine
- 2 tbsp. butter; melted
- 2 gold potatoes; cubed

- Salt and black pepper to taste

Directions:

1. Season the duck pieces with salt and pepper, put them in a pan and heat up over medium-high heat.

2. Cook for 4 minutes on each side, transfer to your air fryer's basket and cook at 360°F for 8 minutes

3. Put the butter in a pan and heat it up over medium heat; then add the potatoes, salt, pepper and the wine and cook for 8 minutes

4. Add the duck pieces, toss and cook everything for 3-4 minutes more. Divide all between plates and serve.

Chicken and Chickpeas

Preparation Time: 35 minutes

Servings: 4

Ingredients:

- 2 lbs. chicken thighs; boneless
- 8 oz. canned chickpeas; drained
- 5 oz. bacon; cooked and crumbled
- 1 cup chicken stock
- 1 tsp. balsamic v*inegar
- 2 tbsp. olive oil
- 1 cup yellow onion; chopped.
- 2 carrots; chopped.
- 1 tbsp. parsley; chopped.
- Salt and black pepper to taste

Directions:

1. Heat up a pan that fits your air fryer with the oil over medium heat.
2. Add the onions, carrots, salt and pepper; stir and sauté for 3-4 minutes.

3. Add the chicken, stock, vinegar and chickpeas; then toss

4. Place the pan in the fryer and cook at 380°F for 20 minutes

5. Add the bacon and the parsley and toss again. Divide everything between plates and serve.

Honey Mustard Cheesy Meatballs

Preparation Time: 15 minutes

Cooking Time: 15 minutes

Servings: 8

Ingredients:

- 2 onions, chopped
- 1 pound ground beef
- 4 tablespoons fresh basil, chopped
- 2 tablespoons cheddar cheese, grated
- 2 teaspoons garlic paste
- 2 teaspoons honey
- Salt and black pepper, to taste
- 2 teaspoons mustard

Directions:

1. Preheat the Air fryer to 385^{0}F and grease an Air fryer basket.
2. Mix all the ingredients in a bowl until well combined.
3. Shape the mixture into equal-sized balls gently

and arrange the meatballs in the Air fryer basket.

4. Cook for about 15 minutes and dish out to serve warm.

Nutrition:

Calories: 134, Fat: 4.4g, Carbohydrates: 4.6g, Sugar: 2.7g, Protein: 18.2g, Sodium: 50mg

Spicy Lamb Kebabs

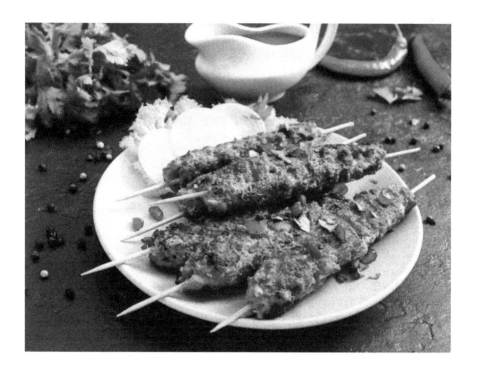

Preparation Time: 20 minutes

Cooking Time: 8 minutes

Servings: 6

Ingredients:

- 4 eggs, beaten
- 1 cup pistachios, chopped

- 1 pound ground lamb

- 4 tablespoons plain flour

- 4 tablespoons flat-leaf parsley, chopped

- 2 teaspoons chili flakes

- 4 garlic cloves, minced

- 2 tablespoons fresh lemon juice

- 2 teaspoons cumin seeds

- 1 teaspoon fennel seeds

- 2 teaspoons dried mint

- 2 teaspoons salt

- Olive oil

- 1 teaspoon coriander seeds

- 1 teaspoon freshly ground black pepper

Directions:

1. Preheat the Air fryer to 355 degree F and grease an Air fryer basket.

2. Mix lamb, pistachios, eggs, lemon juice, chili flakes, flour, cumin seeds, fennel seeds, coriander seeds, mint, parsley, salt and black pepper in a large bowl.

3. Thread the lamb mixture onto metal skewers to

form sausages and coat with olive oil.

4. Place the skewers in the Air fryer basket and cook for about 8 minutes.

5. Dish out in a platter and serve hot.

Nutrition:

Calories: 284, Fat: 15.8g, Carbohydrates: 8.4g, Sugar: 1.1g, Protein: 27.9g, Sodium: 932mg

Lamb with Potatoes

Preparation Time: 20 minutes

Cooking Time: 15 minutes

Servings: 2

Ingredients:

- ½ pound lamb meat
- 2 small potatoes, peeled and halved
- ½ small onion, peeled and halved
- ¼ cup frozen sweet potato fries
- 1 garlic clove, crushed
- ½ tablespoon dried rosemary, crushed
- 1 teaspoon olive oil

Directions:

1. Preheat the Air fryer to 355 degree F and arrange a divider in the Air fryer.
2. Rub the lamb evenly with garlic and rosemary and place on one side of Air fryer divider.
3. Cook for about 20 minutes and meanwhile, microwave the potatoes for about 4 minutes.

4. Dish out the potatoes in a large bowl and stir in the olive oil and onions.

5. Transfer into the Air fryer divider and change the side of lamb ramp.

6. Cook for about 15 minutes, flipping once in between and dish out in a bowl.

Nutrition:

Calories: 399, Fat: 18.5g, Carbohydrates: 32.3g, Sugar: 3.8g, Protein: 24.5g, Sodium: 104mg

Italian Beef Meatballs

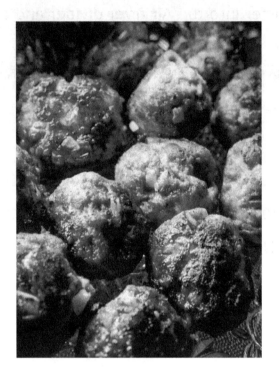

Preparation Time: 10 minutes

Cooking Time: 15 minutes

Servings: 6

Ingredients:

- 2 large eggs
- 2 pounds ground beef

- ¼ cup fresh parsley, chopped
- 1¼ cups panko breadcrumbs
- ¼ cup Parmigiano Reggiano, grated
- 1 teaspoon dried oregano
- 1 small garlic clove, chopped
- Salt and black pepper, to taste
- 1 teaspoon vegetable oil

Directions:

1. Preheat the Air fryer to 350 degree F and grease an Air fryer basket.
2. Mix beef with all other ingredients in a bowl until well combined.
3. Make equal-sized balls from the mixture and arrange the balls in the Air fryer basket.
4. Cook for about 13 minutes and dish out to serve warm.

Nutrition:

Calories: 398, Fat: 13.8g, Carbohydrates: 3.6g, Sugar: 1.3g, Protein: 51.8g, Sodium: 272mg

Pork Chops with Chicory Treviso

Preparation time: 10-20;

Cooking time: 0-15;

Serve: 2

Ingredients:

- 4 pork chops
- 40g butter
- Flour to taste
- 1 chicory stalk
- Salt to taste

Directions:

1. Cut the chicory into small pieces. Place the butter and chicory in pieces on the basket of the air fryer previously preheated at 180°C and brown for 2 min.

2. Add the previously floured and salted pork slices (directly over the chicory), simmer for 6 minutes turning them over after 3 minutes.

3. Remove the slices and place them on a serving

plate, covering them with the rest of the red chicory juice collected at the bottom of the basket.

Nutrition:

Calories 504, Fat 33, Carbohydrates 0g, Sugars 0g, Protein 42g, Cholesterol 130mg

Pork Chops and Spinach

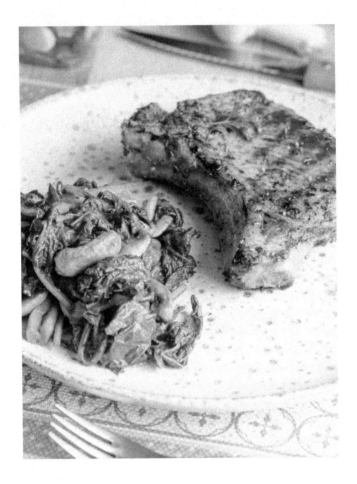

Preparation Time: 20 minutes

Servings: 4

Ingredients:

- 2 pork chops
- 1/4 cup beef stock
- 3 tbsp. spinach pesto
- 2 cups baby spinach
- Salt and black pepper to taste

Directions:

1. Place the pork chops, salt, pepper and spinach pesto in a bowl; toss well
2. Place the pork chops in the air fryer and cook at 400°F for 4 minutes on each side.
3. Transfer the chops to a pan that fits your air fryer and add the stock and the baby spinach
4. Put the pan in the fryer and cook at 400°F for 7 minutes more. Divide everything between plates and serve.

Lamb Ribs

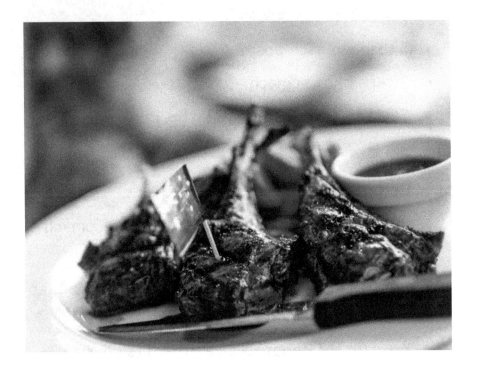

Preparation Time: 20 minutes

Servings: 4

Ingredients:

- 4 lamb ribs
- 1 cup veggie stock
- 1/4 tsp. smoked paprika

- 1/2 tsp. chili powder

- 2 tbsp. extra virgin olive oil

- 4 garlic cloves; minced

- Salt and black pepper to taste

Directions:

1. In a bowl; combine all of the ingredients except the ribs and mix well.

2. Then add the ribs and rub them thoroughly with the mixture

3. Transfer the ribs to your air fryer's basket and cook at 390°F for 7 minutes on each side. Serve with a side salad

Basil Beef Roast

Preparation Time: 60 minutes

Servings: 6

Ingredients:

- 1½ lbs. beef roast
- 2 garlic cloves; minced
- 1 cup beef stock
- 2 carrots; sliced
- 1 tbsp. basil; dried
- Salt and black pepper to taste

Directions:

1. In a pan that fits your air fryer, combine all ingredients well.
2. Place the pan in the fryer and cook at 390°F for 55 minutes
3. Slice the roast, divide it and the carrots between plates and serve with cooking juices drizzled on top.

Glazed Ham

Servings: 4

Preparation Time: 15 minutes

Cooking Time: 40 minutes

Ingredients

- 1 pound 10½ ounces ham
- 1 cup whiskey
- 2 tablespoons French mustard
- 2 tablespoons honey

Directions:

1. Place the ham at room temperature for about 30 minutes before cooking.

2. In a bowl, mix together the whiskey, mustard, and honey.

3. Place the ham in a baking dish that fits in the air fryer.

4. Top with half of the honey mixture and coat well.

5. Set the temperature of air fryer to 320 degrees F. Place the baking dish into the air

fryer.

6.   Air fry for about 15 minutes.

7.   Flip the side of ham and top with the remaining honey mixture.

8.   Air fry for about 25 more minutes.

9.   Remove from air fryer and place the ham onto a platter for about 10 minutes before slicing.

10. Cut the ham into desired size slices and serve.

Nutrition:

Calories: 558, Carbohydrate: 18.6g, Protein: 43g, Fat: 22.2g, Sugar: 8.7g, Sodium: 3000mg

Peanut Butter Cookies

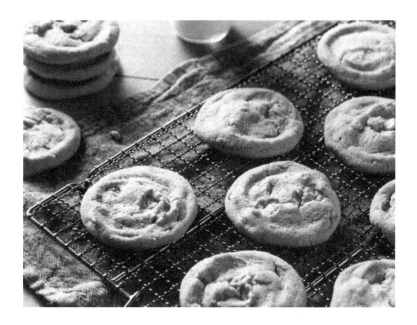

Preparation Time: 13 minutes

Servings: 8

Ingredients:

- 1 large egg.
- ⅓ cup granular erythritol.
- 1 cup no-sugar-added smooth peanut butter.
- 1 tsp. vanilla extract.

Directions:

1. Take a large bowl, mix all ingredients until smooth. Continue stirring for 2 additional minutes and the mixture will begin to thicken.
2. Roll the mixture into eight balls and press gently down to flatten into 2-inch round disks.
3. Cut a piece of parchment to fit your air fryer and place it into the basket. Place the cookies onto the parchment, working in batches as necessary.
4. Adjust the temperature to 320 Degrees F and set the timer for 8 minutes.
5. Flip the cookies at the 6-minute mark. Serve completely cooled.

Nutrition:

Calories: 210; Protein: 8.8g; Fiber: 2.0g; Fat: 17.5g; Carbs: 14.1g

Kale and Brussels Sprouts

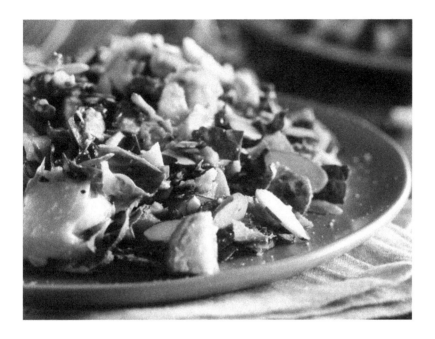

Preparation Time: 20 minutes

Servings: 8

Ingredients:

- 1 lb. Brussels sprouts, trimmed
- 3 oz. mozzarella, shredded
- 2 cups kale, torn
- 1 tbsp. olive oil

- Salt and black pepper to taste.

Directions:

1. In a pan that fits the air fryer, combine all the Ingredients: except the mozzarella and toss.
2. Put the pan in the air fryer and cook at 380°F for 15 minutes
3. Divide between plates, sprinkle the cheese on top and serve.

Nutrition:

Calories: 170; Fat: 5g; Fiber: 3g; Carbs: 4g; Protein: 7g

Zucchini and Olives

Preparation Time: 17 minutes

Servings: 4

Ingredients

- 4 zucchinis; sliced
- 2 tbsp. olive oil
- 1 cup kalamata olives, pitted
- 2 tbsp. lime juice
- 2 tsp. balsamic vinegar
- Salt and black pepper to taste.

Directions:

1. In a pan that fits your air fryer, mix the olives with all the other Ingredients:, toss, introduce in the fryer and cook at 390°F for 12 minutes
2. Divide the mix between plates and serve.

Nutrition:

Calories: 150; Fat: 4g; Fiber: 2g; Carbs: 4g; Protein: 5g

Sweet & Spicy Parsnips

Servings: 6

Preparation Time: 15 minutes

Cooking Time: 44 minutes

Ingredients

- 2 pounds parsnip, peeled and cut into 1-inch chunks
- 1 tablespoon butter, melted
- 2 tablespoons honey
- 1 tablespoon dried parsley flakes, crushed
- ¼ teaspoon red pepper flakes, crushed
- Salt and ground black pepper, as required

Directions:

1. Set the temperature of air fryer to 355 degrees F. Grease an air fryer basket.

2. In a large bowl, mix together the parsnips and butter.

3. Arrange parsnip chunks into the prepared air

fryer basket in a single layer.

4. Air fry for about 40 minutes.

5. Meanwhile, in another large bowl, mix well remaining ingredients.

6. After 40 minutes, transfer parsnips into the bowl of honey mixture and toss to coat well.

7. Again, arrange the parsnip chunks into air fryer basket in a single layer.

8. Air fry for 3-4 more minutes.

9. Remove from air fryer and transfer the parsnip chunks onto serving plates.

10. Serve hot.

Nutrition:

Calories: 155, Carbohydrate: 33.1g, Protein: 1.9g, Fat: 2.4g, Sugar: 13g, Sodium: 57mg

Green Chicken Chili

Preparation Time: 10 minutes

Cooking Time: 35 minutes

Servings: 8

Ingredients:

- 2 tbsp. unsalted butter
- 1 medium yellow onion (to be peeled and chopped)
- ½ lb. poblano peppers (to be seeded and roughly chopped)
- ½ lb. Anaheim peppers (to be seeded and roughly chopped)
- ½ lb. tomatillos (to be husked and quartered)
- 2 small jalapeño peppers (to be seeded and roughly chopped)
- 2 garlic cloves (to be peeled and minced)
- 1 tsp. ground cumin
- 6 bone-in, skin-on chicken thighs (2 ½ lbs. in total)
- 2 cups chicken stock

- 2 cups water

- 1/3 cup roughly chopped fresh cilantro

- 3 cans Great Northern beans (to be drained and rinsed, 15 oz. cans)

Directions:

1. Choose the "Sauté" button on the Air fryer and when hot, add butter to melt. Once the butter melts, add onion and cook for about 3 minutes until softened. Add poblano and Anaheim peppers, then tomatillos, and jalapeños. Cook 3 minutes add garlic and cumin. Cook about 30 seconds or until fragrant. Then cancel sautéing.

2. Add the thighs, stock, and water to pot and stir. Tightly close lid and have the steam release set to the "Sealing" position. Select the "Rice/Grain" option and set the timer for 30 minutes. At the end of the cook time, do a quick release of pressure and open lid to stir well. Press the "Cancel" button and transfer the chicken to a cutting board. After carefully removing the skin, shred the meat with two forks.

3. Using an immersion blender, purée the sauce

until smooth. Stir in the meat, cilantro, and beans and serve warm.

Nutrition:

Calories – 304 Protein – 33 g. Fat – 10 g. Carbs – 19 g.

Crushed Lentil Soup

Preparation Time: 10 minutes

Cooking Time: 30 minutes

Servings: 8

Ingredients:

- 2 tablespoons vegetable broth
- 1 onion, finely chopped
- 4 garlic cloves, minced
- 4 cups unsalted vegetable broth
- 2 cups of water
- 2 cups red split lentils
- 1 small pinch saffron
- 1 teaspoon coriander
- 1 teaspoon cumin
- ½ teaspoon freshly ground black pepper
- 1 teaspoon sea salt
- ½ teaspoon of red pepper flakes
- 2 bay leaves
- 2 tablespoons fresh lemon juice

Directions:

1. Put the air fryer to saute, add the vegetable broth, 2 tablespoons. Then put in the garlic and onions and cook until they are soft, about 4-5 minutes.

2. Add remaining ingredients except for bay leaves and lemon juice. Stir and then lock the lid of the air fryer.

3. Press cancel and choose the soup function. Set timer for 30 minutes. After the 30 minutes, let it sit for another 20 minutes to release the pressure.

4. Open the lid and add bay leaves and lemon juice, then stir for 5 minutes.

5. Remove bay leaves and serve.

Nutrition:

Calories – 191 Protein – 11.8 g. Fat – 1.2 g. Carbs – 34.4 g.

Carrot Soup with Fowl

Preparation Time: 8 minutes

Cooking Time: 20 minutes

Servings: 4

Ingredients:

- ½ fowl or chicken
- 2 quarts of chicken broth
- ¼ Cup of coarsely chopped onion
- ½ Cup of coarsely chopped carrots
- ½ Cup of coarsely chopped celery
- 1 Teaspoon of saffron threads
- ¾ Cup of corn kernels
- ½ Cup of finely chopped celery
- 1 tablespoon of fresh chopped parsley
- 1 Cup of cooked egg noodles

Directions:

1. Start by combining all together the stewing chicken or fowl with the chicken broth in your Air fryer

2. Press sauté and add the onions, the carrots, the celery and the saffron

3. Now, close the lid and set at high pressure for around 20 minutes

4. Once the timer beeps, remove the chicken and shred it from the bone and cut it into small pieces

5. Strain your saffron broth with a fine sieve and then add the celery, the corn, the parsley, and the cooked noodles to your broth.

6. Return your soup to simmer for a few minutes

7. Serve and enjoy a delicious and nutritious soup

Nutrition:

Calories – 154.4 Protein – 10.9 g. Fat – 0.8 g. Carbs – 27.2 g.

Lemony Lentil Soup

Preparation Time: 10 minutes

Cooking Time: 25 minutes

Servings: 4

Ingredients:

- 1 tablespoon of olive oil
- 1 medium onion, peeled and diced
- 2 carrots, diced
- 5 garlic cloves, minced
- 6 cups of vegetable stock
- 1 1/2 cup of red lentils
- ⅔ cup of whole kernel corn
- 2 teaspoons of ground cumin
- 1 teaspoon of curry powder
- zest and juice of 1 lemon
- sea salt and black pepper to taste

Directions:

1. Choose the saute function on your air fryer and add oil. Add the onions and carrots and saute for

5 minutes. Stir occasionally until the onions are soft and translucent. Add garlic and saute for 1 more minute, until fragrant.

2. Pour in the vegetable stock, lentils, corn, cumin, and curry powder until combined

3. Make sure to lock the lid and set to "sealing."

4. Press and set for manual high pressure, and adjust the timer for 8 minutes. Cook, then carefully turn to venting for quick release. Once vented, remove the lid carefully.

5. Using a blender, puree the soup until it reaches your desired consistency.

6. Return the puree to the air fryer and stir in lemon zest and juice until combined.

7. Season with sea salt and black pepper to taste.

8. Serve warm.

Nutrition:

Calories – 260 Protein – 16 g. Fat – 6 g. Carbs – 40 g.

Manchow Soup

Preparation Time: 10 minutes

Cooking Time: 25 minutes

Servings: 4

Ingredients:

- 3 oz. fried noodles, for garnish
- ½ cup green bell peppers
- ½ cup bean sprouts
- ½ cup mushrooms
- ½ cup broccoli
- ½ cup baby carrots
- 2 green onions, chopped
- 4 garlic cloves, minced
- ½ inch ginger, minced
- 1 teaspoon soy sauce
- 1 teaspoon vinegar
- 2 teaspoons chilli sauce
- 3 cups vegetable stock
- 1 tablespoon oil
- Salt and pepper, to taste

- Roasted crushed peanuts, for garnish

Directions:

1. Put the oil, ginger, garlic, carrots, onions and carrots in the Air fryer and select "Sauté".
2. Sauté for 4 minutes and add soy sauce, chilli sauce, vinegar and vegetable stock.
3. Set the Air fryer to "Soup" and cook for 10 minutes at high pressure.
4. Release the pressure naturally and add cooked noodles.
5. Season with salt and black pepper and garnish with fried noodles and crushed roasted peanuts.

Nutrition:

Calories: 379; Total Fat: 20.8g; Carbs: 43.6g; Sugars: 2.4g; Protein: 8.7g

Air fryer Mediterranean Chicken And Quinoa Stew

Preparation Time: 10 minutes

Cooking Time: 20 minutes

Servings: 6

Ingredients:

- 1-¼ pounds of chicken thighs, boneless and skinless
- 4 cups of butternut squash, peeled and chopped
- 4 cups unsalted chicken stock
- 1 cup yellow onion, chopped
- 2 garlic cloves, chopped
- 1 bay leaf
- 1-¼ teaspoons of kosher salt
- 1 teaspoon of dried oregano
- 1 teaspoon of ground fennel seeds
- ½ cup of uncooked quinoa
- 1-ounce of olives, sliced and pitted

Directions:

1. Combine the chicken, squash, stock, onion, garlic, bay leaf, salt, ground fennel seeds, oregano, and pepper in your air fryer. Cover the lid, turn the valve to seal and cook on high pressure for 8 minutes.

2. Release the valve carefully, using mitts or tongs. Quick-release until the steam and pressure go down. Remove chicken, then add quinoa to the air fryer, turn to saute and cook while occasionally stirring until the quinoa is tender.

3. Shred the chicken and stir into stew. Discard bay leaf.

4. Serve the soup up into separate bowls, and sprinkle sliced olives.

Nutrition:

Calories – 243 Protein – 25 g. Fat – 6 g. Carbs – 24 g.

Spices Stuffed Eggplants (Vegan)

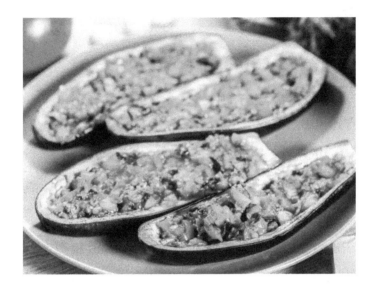

Preparation Time: 15 minutes

Cooking Time: 12 minutes

Servings: 4

Ingredients:

- 8 baby eggplants
- 4 teaspoons olive oil, divided
- ¾ tablespoon dry mango powder
- ¾ tablespoon ground coriander
- ½ teaspoon ground cumin

- ½ teaspoon ground turmeric

- ½ teaspoon garlic powder

- Salt, to taste

Directions:

1. Preheat the Air fryer to 370 degree F and grease an Air fryer basket.

2. Make 2 slits from the bottom of each eggplant leaving the stems intact.

3. Mix one teaspoon of oil and spices in a bowl and fill each slit of eggplants with this mixture.

4. Brush the outer side of each eggplant with remaining oil and arrange in the Air fryer basket.

5. Cook for about 12 minutes and dish out in a serving plate to serve hot.

Nutrition:

Calories: 317, Fats: 6.7g, Carbohydrates: 65g, Sugar: 33g, Proteins: 10.9g, Sodium: 61mg

Basil Tomatoes (Vegan)

Servings: 2

Preparation Time: 10 minutes

Cooking Time: 10 minutes

Ingredients

- 2 tomatoes, halved
- Olive oil cooking spray
- Salt and ground black pepper, as required
- 1 tablespoon fresh basil, chopped

Directions:

1. Set the temperature of air fryer to 320 degrees F. Grease an air fryer basket.
2. Spray the tomato halves evenly with cooking spray and sprinkle with salt, black pepper and basil.
3. Arrange tomato halves into the prepared air fryer basket, cut sides up.
4. Air fry for about 10 minutes or until desired doneness.

5. Remove from air fryer and transfer the tomatoes onto serving plates.

6. Serve warm.

Nutrition:

Calories: 22, Carbohydrate: 4.8g, Protein: 1.1g, Fat: 4.8g, Sugar: 3.2g, Sodium: 84mg

Sweet & Spicy Cauliflower (Vegan)

Servings: 4

Preparation Time: 15 minutes

Cooking Time: 30 minutes

Ingredients

- 1 head cauliflower, cut into florets
- ¾ cup onion, thinly sliced
- 5 garlic cloves, finely sliced
- 1½ tablespoons soy sauce
- 1 tablespoon hot sauce
- 1 tablespoon rice vinegar
- 1 teaspoon coconut sugar
- Pinch of red pepper flakes
- Ground black pepper, as required
- 2 scallions, chopped

Directions:

1. Set the temperature of air fryer to 350 degrees F. Grease an air fryer pan.

2. Arrange cauliflower florets into the prepared

air fryer pan in a single layer.

3. Air fry for about 10 minutes.

4. Remove from air fryer and stir in the onions.

5. Air fry for another 10 minutes.

6. Remove from air fryer and stir in the garlic.

7. Air fry for 5 more minutes.

8. Meanwhile, in a bowl, mix well soy sauce, hot sauce, vinegar, coconut sugar, red pepper flakes, and black pepper.

9. Remove from the air fryer and stir in the sauce mixture.

10. Air fry for about 5 minutes.

11. Remove from air fryer and transfer the cauliflower mixture onto serving plates.

12. Garnish with scallions and serve.

Nutrition:

Calories: 72, Carbohydrate: 13.8g, Protein: 3.6g, Fat: 0.2g, Sugar: 3.1g, Sodium: 1300mg

Herbed Potatoes (Vegan)

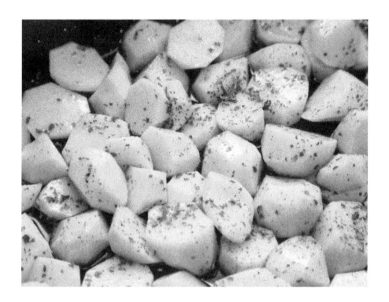

Servings: 4

Preparation Time: 10 minutes

Cooking Time: 16 minutes

Ingredients

- 6 small potatoes, chopped
- 3 tablespoons olive oil
- 2 teaspoons mixed dried herbs
- Salt and ground black pepper, as required

- 2 tablespoons fresh parsley, chopped

Directions:

1. Set the temperature of air fryer to 356 degrees F. Grease an air fryer basket.
2. In a large bowl, add the potatoes, oil, herbs, salt and black pepper and toss to coat well.
3. Arrange the chopped potatoes into the prepared air fryer basket in a single layer.
4. Air fry for about 16 minutes, tossing once halfway through.
5. Remove from air fryer and transfer the potatoes onto serving plates.
6. Garnish with parsley and serve.

Nutrition:

Calories: 268, Carbohydrate: 40.4g, Protein: 4.4g, Fat: 10.8g, Sugar: 3g, Sodium: 55mg

Jalapeño Bacon Cheese Bread

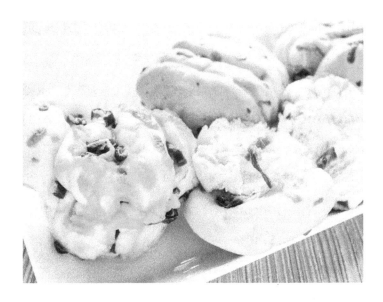

Preparation Time: 25 minutes

Servings: 8 sticks

Ingredients:

- 4 slices sugar-free bacon; cooked and chopped
- 2 large eggs.
- ¼ cup chopped pickled jalapeños.
- ¼ cup grated Parmesan cheese.
- 2 cups shredded mozzarella cheese

Directions:

1. Mix all ingredients in a large bowl. Cut a piece of parchment to fit your air fryer basket.

2. Dampen your hands with a bit of water and press out the mixture into a circle. You may need to separate this into two smaller cheese breads, depending on the size of your fryer

3. Place the parchment and cheese bread into the air fryer basket

4. Adjust the temperature to 320 Degrees F and set the timer for 15 minutes. Carefully flip the bread when 5 minutes remain

5. When fully cooked, the top will be golden brown. Serve warm.

Nutrition:

Calories: 273; Protein: 20.1g; Fiber: 0.1g; Fat: 18.1g; Carbs: 2.3g

Apple Doughnuts

Preparation Time: 20 minutes

Cooking Time: 5 minutes

Servings: 6

Ingredients:

- 2½ cups plus 2 tablespoons all-purpose flour
- 1½ teaspoons baking powder
- 2 tablespoons unsalted butter, softened
- 1 egg
- ½ pink lady apple, peeled, cored and grated
- 1 cup apple cider
- ½ teaspoon ground cinnamon
- ½ teaspoon salt
- ½ cup brown sugar

Directions:

1. Preheat the Air fryer to 360 degree F and grease an Air fryer basket lightly.
2. Boil apple cider in a medium pan over medium-high heat and reduce the heat.

3. Let it simmer for about 15 minutes and dish out in a bowl.

4. Sift together flour, baking powder, baking soda, cinnamon, and salt in a large bowl.

5. Mix the brown sugar, egg, cooled apple cider and butter in another bowl.

6. Stir in the flour mixture and grated apple and mix to form a dough.

7. Wrap the dough with a plastic wrap and refrigerate for about 30 minutes.

8. Roll the dough into 1-inch thickness and cut the doughnuts with a doughnut cutter.

9. Arrange the doughnuts into the Air fryer basket and cook for about 5 minutes, flipping once in between.

10. Dish out and serve warm.

Nutrition:

Calories: 433, Fat: 11g, Carbohydrates: 78.3g, Sugar: 35g, Protein: 6.8g, Sodium: 383mg

Lemon Cake

Preparation Time: 22 minutes

Servings: 6

Ingredients:

- 3 oz. brown sugar
- 3 oz. flour
- 1 tsp. dark chocolate; grated
- 3½ oz. butter; melted
- 3 eggs
- 1/2 tsp. lemon juice

Directions:

1. Mix all of the ingredients in a bowl.
2. Pour the mixture into a greased cake pan and place in the fryer
3. Cook at 360°F for 17 minutes. Let cake cool before serving

Butter Donuts

Preparation Time: 25 minutes

Servings: 4

Ingredients:

- 8 oz. flour
- 4 oz. whole milk
- 1 egg
- 2½ tbsp. butter
- 1 tbsp. brown sugar
- 1 tbsp. white sugar
- 1 tsp. baking powder

Directions:

1. Place all of the ingredients in a bowl and mix well.
2. Shape donuts from this mix and place them in your air fryer's basket
3. Cook at 360°F for 15 minutes. Arrange the donuts on a platter and serve them warm

Chocolate Pudding

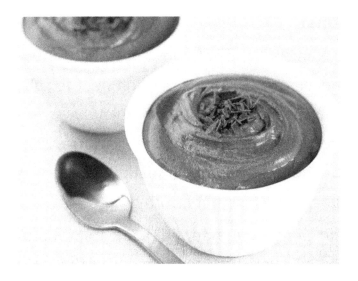

Preparation Time: 34 minutes

Servings: 4

Ingredients:

- 1/4 cup fresh orange juice
- 2/3 cup dark chocolate; chopped
- 1/2 cup butter
- 1/4 cup caster sugar
- 2 medium eggs
- 2 tbsp. self-rising flour

- 2 tsp. fresh orange rind, finely grated

Directions:

1. In a microwave-safe bowl; add the butter and chocolate. Microwave on high heat for about 2 minutes or until melted completely, stirring after every 30 seconds. Remove from microwave and stir the mixture until smooth. Add the sugar and eggs and whisk until frothy

2. Add the orange rind and juice, followed by flour and mix until well combined. Set the temperature of air fryer to 355°F. Grease 4 ramekins.

3. Divide mixture into the prepared ramekins about ¾ full. Air fry for about 12 minutes

4. Remove from the air fryer and set aside to completely cool before serving. Serve warm

Brioche Pudding

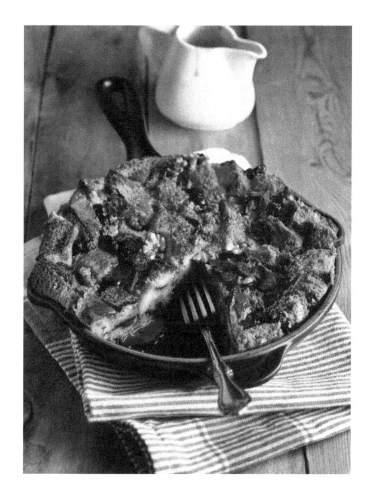

Preparation Time: 35 minutes

Servings: 4

Ingredients:

- 3 cups brioche; cubed
- 2 cups half and half
- 2 cups milk
- 1/2 tsp. vanilla extract
- 1/2 cup raisins
- 1 cup sugar
- 4 egg yolks; whisked
- 2 tbsp. butter; melted
- Zest of 1/2 lemon

Directions:

1. In a bowl, add all of the ingredients and whisk well
2. Pour the mixture into a pudding mould and place it in the air fryer
3. Cook at 330°F for 30 minutes. Cool down and serve.

Lemon Chocolate Cookies

Servings: 4

Preparation Time: 15 minutes

Cooking Time: 5 minutes

Ingredients:

- 1 cup almond flour
- 6 tablespoons butter
- 4 tablespoons Stevia
- 1 egg yolk
- ½ cup semi-sweet chocolate chips

Directions

1. Place butter and stevia in a mixing bowl then using an electric mixer beat until fluffy.
2. Add egg yolk to the bowl then continue beating until incorporated.
3. Stir almond flour into the mixture then using a wooden spatula mix until becoming dough.
4. Add chocolate chips to the dough then mix until just combined.

5. Preheat an Air Fryer to 180°F (82°C).

6. Shape the dough into small ball forms then arrange in the Air Fryer.

7. Press the cookie balls until becoming coin forms then cook in the Air Fryer for 5 minutes.

8. Once it is done, remove from the Air Fryer then place on a cooling rack. Let them cool.

9. Serve and enjoy.

Nutrition Values:

Net Carbs: 5.4g; Calories: 246; Total Fat: 23.9g; Saturated Fat: 12.6g

Protein: 2.9g; Carbs: 6.7g

Notes